Stretching

Stretching Exercises for Beginners

—

Quick Ways to Become Flexible and Gain Strength

Dan C. Wilson

© 2015

Table of Contents

About the Author

Other Books by Dan C. Wilson

Introduction

I would like to thank you for downloading this book about stretching exercises for beginners. You will find many answers to your questions about how to stretch properly, how to avoid injuries and how to improve your muscle flexibility. I would like to encourage you to practice, repeat and re-read this book as many times as needed to fully understand the content about flexibility training.

Everything I know about sports, training and nutrition, I learned from the best training mentors as well as my own research and experience. I got taught the most modern methods of training. I am grateful to all my mentors for bringing the importance of physical education and sports to the attention of me, which allows me to pass on this information to you.

It is a body of knowledge that makes all the difference between success and failure in developing athletic skills and abilities, or simply in getting results from exercises. In describing the methods of stretching, I have given as much information about the correct ways of working out as possible without making this book an advanced manual about physical education and sports training. All the information you find in this book is through own experience and the methodology of my mentors.

This book will give you all the information you need to accomplish the maximum flexibility permitted by your body structure and flexibility training you may need for your sport. Simultaneous it will also develop your strength by the use of heavy stretching's. You will learn to work with your body for full flexibility.

Dan C. Wilson

Chapter 1: Benefits of Stretching

Before we get straight down to the exercises, it is important to understand the benefits of stretching and why we should use them more often in our daily life. Any movement you make that requires moving a body part to the point at which there is an increase in the movement of a joint can be called a stretching exercise. There are many benefits gained from using a regular stretching program. I have listed down below some of the benefits of stretching for you.

- ✓ Good muscular and joint mobility.
- ✓ Improved appearance and self-image.
- ✓ Reduced injuries and pains – Use light stretches if the pain prevails.
- ✓ Improved muscular strength, flexibility and stamina – The benefit depends on the degree of how much stress you put on your muscle. For gaining more strength, medium or heavy stretches are recommended. Further in this book we will examine light, medium and heavy stretching.
- ✓ Improved body alignment and posture.

✓ Prevention of back problems.

Good flexibility is known to bring positive benefits in the muscles and joints. It aids with injury prevention and helps you to minimize muscle pains. Efficiency in all physical activities will be improved and increasing flexibility will also improve quality of life as well as functional independence. Good flexibility improves the elasticity of your muscles and provides a wider range of motion in the joints. Ease in body movements will be provided for your everyday activities. A simple daily task such as bending over and tying shoes is accomplished better with flexibility.

For every person, whether you are an athlete or not, a regular basic stretching program can bring some great benefits to you. Recent research studies on various injuries have shown that people with low flexibility have a highly increased chance of muscle injuries. However, the type of flexibility needed for reducing those injuries did not come from doing stretching exercises right before the activity as a warm-up. The flexibility required for a lower chance of getting injuries came from following a stretch training for a certain amount of weeks. Increased strength and endurance gains have been reported as well as improved flexibility and mobility.

A few general tips for when you are about to do your stretching exercises, try to include all the major muscle groups in your program. It is highly recommended to do at least two different stretches for each joint movement. In case you are about to start with a physical activity, use light stretches as part of your warm-up.

Once you are done with your exercise routine, cool down with light- or medium-intensity stretches. Should your muscles be sore after your exercises, try to use only light stretches ranging from two to three times. Should your muscle soreness or injury persist for several days, then I recommend to continue using light stretches only. It is very important to give your muscles enough rest to recover, instead of forcing it.

1.1
Know Your Limits

Now that we know the many great benefits that stretching has to offer, it is also important to know your limits and what to avoid. Firstly, we will focus on the first step of any workout program. Knowing your limits. A workout should be something that you enjoy and look forward to, it should be a pleasurable part of your day. It can be the first thing you do in the morning when you wake up, or in the evening when you finished your working shift. There may be times you experience some muscle soreness while working out or after a workout, however, it should not be the type of pain that interferes with your functional behavior. The same theory goes for stretching. Stretching properly before, during and after a workout session, you will definitely decrease the chances of obtaining some serious injuries and you will avoid muscle soreness and pains.

It is therefore extremely important to know your body limits. Stretching is an activity that should improve your body stamina, rather than causing you pain. Stretching was invented to avoid pain and become more flexible. It might happen that you feel a small mild tension when you stretch, do not worry as this is just a temporary feeling from your body stiffness. In case you do feel any pain beyond the stiffness, you have gone too far and you should lower the tense level of your stretching.

Should you feel pain during stretching, this means that your body has employed its defense mechanism – the stretch reflex. This happens when you stretch your muscles and tendons to the point of pain. Your body has a safety measure to prevent some serious damage caused to the muscles and tendons. The stretch reflex is a protection of your muscles and tendons and prevents them from being stretched beyond their possible limits. Do never try to force your body beyond this protection point. You will risk causing serious damage to your muscle tissues, tendons and ligaments.

1.2
Things to Avoid

Stretching is one of the most underutilized techniques for improving athletic performance, preventing sports injury and properly rehabilitating muscle injuries. Most people have never learnt the proper way of stretching. By nature we often copy the behavior of other people unconsciously, this happens in the gym as well when you watch other people stretching and you then try to imitate what they are doing. Rarely people ask themselves if they are doing it the right way. Do not make the mistake of thinking that something as simple as stretching will not be effective. We will now examine the most common mistakes while stretching.

Bouncing
This is a very dangerous movement as this will often lead to the edge of your stretch reflex, explained earlier. People often mistake the impression that they should bounce to get a good stretch. However, this will usually do more damage than harm to you as you try to push your body limits too far. Every physical move you make during a workout or while stretching should be smooth and gentle. Gradually lean into the stretch and push to the point of very mild tension. Once your muscles have loosened up, you will be able

to go a little bit further. Make sure to not force or overdo it.

Stretching time period
A common mistake is to not hold the stretch long enough. People get impatient and try to rush through the stretch workout or do not hold the stretch long enough, often this also results in the habit of bouncing. A rule of thumb is to hold your stretch position for at least 15 to 25 seconds before you move back to your original position.

High training load
Spending every day hours in the gym will result in a wrong training load, which will be too great without enough rest and eventually this will cause chronic fatigue. If you begin your workout still sore after the previous one, you are asking for an injury or at least you hamper your further progress. Always make sure to have enough rest between your physical activities.

Stretching too tense
Understand that stretching takes patience and finesse. Every move that you make needs to be fluid and gentle. Try to avoid throwing your body into a stretch or trying to rush through your stretching movements. It is recommended to take your time to make sure that the movements are done correctly.

Incorrect form and function

A very helpful tip is to think about your physical activity before you start stretching. Which muscles are you going to use? It is important to know which muscles you are about to use, an athlete who is going to run a couple of miles will be using different muscles compared to a person who is planning to do an hour of weights lifting. Carefully pay attention to the muscles you have to use in your workout program, and also make sure to attain and maintain the correct form for each stretch. Consider the range of motion you are going to put through the particular muscle. The reason why we stretch is to get our muscles accustomed to move through a specific range of motion. Always try to think about which muscles you will be using and how.

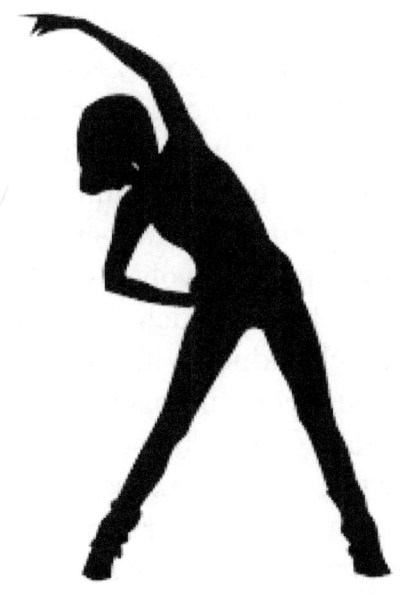

Chapter 2: Stretching Methods

Knowing the right stretching method is a great asset to have as this will allow you to have great flexibility even without a warm-up. It is essential for especially athletes to have such flexibility so they can demonstrate a technique immediately when it is needed. Lacking this ability will indicate that either the use of your stretching method is incorrect or you are chronically fatigued. In some cases it indicates that you are currently dealing with both scenarios.

Should you be one of the persons who have this flexibility, bare in mind to not to get too confident. In case you are familiar and experienced with sports, you will not necessarily always have to do a full set of stretching before doing a few full range of motion moves without a warm-up, however you should never overdo it. Many sports involve sudden twisting or bending of the trunk, such as football, rugby, basketball and kickboxing. Without warming up your muscles this will result in back pain. The back is wrapped in deep layers of muscles. The more larger and deeper the mass of your muscles are, the longer it takes to warm them up. Warming them up before doing your workout will result in recovery afterwards.

One of the easiest tasks in athletic training is to develop great flexibility. One can reach an exceptional level with very little time and effort. With rational training, your flexibility will improve from day to day. We have examined the most common mistakes which withholds most people who spend days and weeks in the gym, without getting better results.

Applying the methodology which you will find in this book, will improve your results and prevents you from making any of the previously discussed mistakes. If you follow the instructions to the letter, you will have very small chances to obtain muscle injuries and pain.

You will find many methods for improving flexibility out there, I have tried to sum up the safest and most efficient methods for you. Your choice of method or combination of methods will depend on your sport and the shape you are in. I will try to guide you towards the best possible methods for you.

2.1
Dynamic Stretching

One of the very good ways of stretching is dynamic stretching. This is involves moving parts of your body and gradually increasing reach and the speed of your movement – such as arm swings for example. Always perform your exercises in sets of 8 to 10 repetitions. Should you feel tired after a few sets, stop immediately. Fatigue will cause a decrease in the amplitude of your movements. It is recommended to only exercise the number of repetitions that you can do without diminishing your range of motion. If you do more repetitions than your body allows, you will more than likely lose some of your flexibility. After you have reached the maximum range of motion in a joint you should stop with this particular movement in a direction. Even if you can maintain your current maximum range of motion, it is not advised to force it.

Dynamic stretches are often confused with static stretches. Dynamic stretches do not involve stopping and holding your stretched position. Dynamic stretching is supposed to increase your dynamic flexibility. Once your body is in motion, the speed of your movements and range will increase. These results are obtained by practicing dynamic stretches.

Not only is dynamic stretching often confused with static stretches, it is confused with ballistic stretching as well. Ballistic stretches are all about using the momentum of a last moving body or limb to forcibly and abruptly increase the range or speed of the motion. Unlike dynamic and static movements, a ballistic movement cannot be corrected or adjusted once it's started. In many cases ballistic or bounce stretches will result in immediate as well as residual pain.

Now that you have learned the differences, you will probably understand that dynamic stretching is very different from ballistic or static stretching. There are no bobbling, bouncing or jerky movements with dynamic stretching. The movements are controlled thoroughly even though they can be quite fast. As opposed to ballistic stretching, the dynamic stretches are not sudden and abrupt.

The arm swings, which we have used previously as an example, can practically be performed with control through the whole range of movement or with no control over a substantial part of the movement as soon as the stretch takes place.

2.2
Static Stretching

Most people who read this are most likely aware of what static stretching is. It involves moving your body into a stretch and then holding it there through the tension of your muscles. You may notice when you tense your muscles harder, you will feel less resistance from your stretched muscles.

There is a difference between doing static active stretches, and passive stretches. Passive stretching involves relaxing your body into a stretch and holding it there by your body weight or by external weights. Interesting to know is, that this type of stretching can be more effective than dynamic stretching for increasing your passive range of motion and decreasing the amount of force needed for your static position.

A very good way to use passive stretches is to relieve cramps of overstimulated muscles. If you have spasms occurring in your muscles that are recovering after an injury or soreness, then you should also be using mainly static stretches. However, should you have sore muscles at that particular time, you may further damage them. When your muscles feel sore, it is a sign to give them rest as you have most likely used them actively. It is very important to find the right balance to not risk any injury which could have been avoided by giving the muscles enough rest. Should you not be entirely sure whether your muscles are sore or not, a safe method is to stretch very lightly.

Always keep in mind that you should not be exercising or stretching after or while being injured. It is advised to wait until you have healed sufficiently and in case you are dealing with a serious injury, you should ask for advice from your doctor.

The most effective duration of passive relaxed stretches is 30 seconds, try to maintain a frequency of once per day. Not more and not less, unless you have a muscle injury or muscle soreness – then I would advise to take more rest as needed.

2.3
Isometric Stretching

Last but not least, we will get more involved with isometric stretching. Doing static stretching alone, will not guarantee an increase of dynamic flexibility equal to the increase of static flexibility. It is therefore important to also understand isometric stretching and use them whenever possible.

While your muscles are fatigued, it may happen that your static flexibility will increase. Therefore, it is a good idea to do your static stretching at the end of the workout. However, isometric stretching is surely the fastest way to develop your passive flexibility. Not only will it improve that, it also improves active flexibility together with strength in various actions. In case you are a young reader, then it is not recommended to do isometric stretching. You should wait until your bones are not growing anymore, and when your muscles are healthy and strong enough to use isometric stretching. The last sentence is also important for the people who have neglected strength training, or were doing it incorrectly. Isometric stretches may harm your muscles and cause injury.

I cannot stress this enough, if you are not ready for isometric stretching and your muscles are very weak, due to neglecting strength training, improper workouts, or stretched with too much force, you should NOT be using isometric stretches. Your muscles can become excessively damaged. Depending on the strength of the muscle or the amount of stress, the damage can announce itself as muscle soreness, or it can announce in very serious muscle damage.

Should this person be you, then start first by making your muscles stronger, I would recommend doing strength exercises with light resistance and a high number of repetitions. Try to do these exercises as slowly as possible and make full stops at the beginning and at the end of each movement. Suggested is to do these exercises at least 3 times with at least 30 repetitions. Aim for exercising the muscles that have the highest chance to be overstretched during your normal workout program.

Normally strength workouts for a given muscle group should be done ideally two to three times per week. Do take not that the amount of strength exercises also depends on your body and muscle reaction to them. In case you have done leg exercises, and your muscles are sore the next day after the strength workout, that means you have exercised too often or too much. Vice versa this also goes for not getting muscle soreness together with poor progress, this means that you should exercise a bit more often or increase the weights.

Do not be afraid to make mistakes, be self-observant. The only way to learn how much and often you can increase your resistance, the frequency of your workout without getting sore muscles, is by trial and error. Muscle soreness means that you have currently lost some of your strength and your muscles are slightly shortened, the soreness is usually the highest on the second day after the overly strenuous workout program. In case you exercise on a rigid schedule such as every other day, despite being sore after the previous workout, you may see your flexibility getting progressively worse rather than better as well.

It can be somewhat difficult to state how long exactly you need to perform light repetition exercises after having found out that your muscles are too sore for isometric stretching. A good way to find this out is to periodically test the reaction of your muscles to isometric stretches. Should they get sore, that means they are still too weak for it.

Next up, I will explain three different methods of doing isometric stretches.

First method

Stretch the muscles and wait a couple of seconds until the mechanism regulating the length of the muscles and tension will readjust. As soon as the mechanism has readjusted the length and tension, increase the stretch and wait again for further readjustments. Repeat this step until you reach the point where you cannot stretch any more. Once you have reached that point, you should apply short strong tensions, followed by quick relaxations and immediate stretches to exceed the limitation point. Try to hold the last tension at least 30 seconds and preferably longer.

Second method

By using the second method you should stretch as much as you can and tense the stretched muscles, hold this stretched and tensed position until you get muscle spasms. When your muscle starts to spasm, decrease the stretch for a moment. Once the spasms stopped, increase and tense your muscles again until you reach the spasms. Important is to hold the last tension for at least 5 minutes.

Third method

The third and last method is the one I have used the most to get the best results. Stretch the muscles and then tense for 3 to 5 seconds, followed by a short moment of relaxation. I recommend staying in the preferred time period of 1 to 5 seconds, and then stretching the muscle again. Prior to stretching, try to maximally tense the muscles whom are about to be stretched for a couple of seconds, followed by a relaxation of 1 to 5 seconds, then stretch the muscles again. When you hit the near maximal stretch, tense again for a couple of seconds to trigger the lower resistance to a stretch and the stretch reflex. Now try and stretch further until you cannot increase the stretch any more.

It is a non-stop experiment to find out what duration and strength you would need of the tension which gives you the best and most stretch upon relaxation. Suggested for the best effects during a stretch is to tense the muscles opposing the stretched ones. Bare in mind that this suggestion cannot be done for every stretch, such as standing stretches for the legs.

Slow and steady, try to increase the time of the last tension to about 30 seconds after several weeks of working out. Recommended is to take a minute of rest when you have reached the 30 seconds goal, and repeat the same stretch again. Try to repeat this 3 to 5 times of a whole stretch per workout.

With the previously described methods, it is important to concentrate on the strength gains in a stretched position. As soon as you cannot increase the stretch, try to concentrate on tensing harder or longer, ideally try to do both. After a while it will translate into a greater stretch. A simple way to increase the tension of a muscle at any given length, is to put extra weight on it. In case you are doing leg splits, try to not support yourself with the help of your arms.

Whichever method you decide to choose of isometric stretching, when doing the stretches, try to breathe naturally with deep and calm abdominal breaths. Inhale prior to tensing and exhale or hold your breath during the maximal tension. Make sure to inhale at the beginning of relaxation and, if possible, exhale with further relaxation and stretch. Should you tense much longer than your normal exhalation, then it is perfectly fine to inhale and exhale several times during the tension. There are positions where it may not be possible or convenient to exhale while relaxing and to increase the stretch between the tensions. Should you find yourself in this position, then try to inhale during relaxation and stretching.

Choosing the preferred and best isometric stretches which you are about to do will highly depend on the form of the movements in which you need greater range of motion. Which one you should start with will depend on the muscle group that you feel like is the first obstacle for you. There is not really a right or wrong way to start with your individual isometric stretches program. For example, in case you would like to bring your outstretched arms behind your back while holding a stick in a narrow grip, it may happen that the first resistance comes from your elbow flexors. This will tell you that you should stretch your elbow flexors first.

Chapter 3:
Warm Up Routine

A crucial part of every physical activity by sports or fitness training program is warming up your muscles. It should not be underestimated how important it is to have a structured warm up routine to prevent muscle injuries. A quality warm up has a number of important key elements. Those key elements should all work together to minimize the chances of muscle injuries or soreness from any physical activity.

Starting with a good warm up prior to any physical activity has a couple of benefits, where the main purpose is to prepare the body and also your mind for more intense activity. While doing your warm up, your body's core temperature will start increasing together with your body's muscle temperature. By increasing these temperatures you are helping to loosen up your muscles.

Besides increasing your body's core and muscle temperature, an effective warm up will also increase both your heart and respiratory rate. This will increase the blood flow in your veins, which in return increases the delivery of oxygen and nutrients to the working muscles. This will all help to prepare the muscles, tendons and joints for more tense activity. A good way of knowing how to structure your warm up is by keeping in mind what the goals or aims are for an effective warm up.

While structuring your personal warm up routine, it is important to start with the easiest and most gentle activity first. Then you can slowly build upon each part with more energetic activities, until your body is at the physical and mental peak which is needed for your sports session. This state will be your maximum level of body preparation for the physical activity you are about to make, it will also minimize the possibility to damage your muscles which may result in a serious sports injury eventually.

Structuring your warm up to achieve the desired goals, you will need to include four key elements in your program. This will ensure an effective and complete warm up. I have listed the four key elements down below for you.

1) General warm up
2) Static stretching
3) Sports specific warm up
4) Dynamic stretching

Just because you start with a general warm up, doesn't necessarily means it is more important than the others. They are all equally important and none of the key elements should be neglected or done insufficient. The four elements work together to bring the body and mind to your body's physical peak, which ensures your body is fully prepared for the activities to come ahead. As stated before, not only does it prepare your body – it also minimizes the risks of sports injuries.

A common mistake or misconception is the confusion what stretching exactly accomplishes as part of the warm up. This often results in causing most people to abandon the stretching part, as it is not considered to be important enough. As you may have over read it, I wrote it specifically down <u>as part of</u> the warm up. Stretching plays a crucial part of the warm up, but it is not the warm up itself. Just stretching as your warm up is insufficient as this does not put your body at the maximum preparation peak. Always remember to use the four important key elements for an effective warm up, as they work together to minimize the risk of injuries, and will also prepare your body for physical activities.

Chapter 4: Beginners Program

In this chapter I have prescribed a program for beginners to improve your flexibility, strength and endurance. If you are new to stretching, or physical activities in general, try not to make any changes until you are fully involved in a regular stretching program. Keep in mind that changes will not come in a couple of days, improving your physical state takes patience and time.

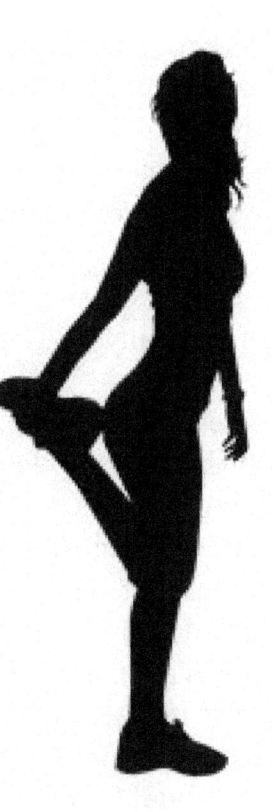

It is perfectly fine should you only be interested in doing daily stretch exercises. To follow this program it is not needed to have another kind of exercise program. Simply by heavy stretching you can already bring changes to your flexibility, strength and endurance. Try not to be overly motivated, make sure that your stretching progression is gradual, moving slowly from a lighter load with a short amount of time spent on each stretch towards a more heavier load with a longer amount of time spent on each stretch.

I have created four easy to follow stretching programs and are based on your initial flexibility. Gradually progress from the first level towards the fourth. Feel free to customize this program according to your current level of experience and flexibility, but do not discard parts of the program. Working through each of the levels with the recommended speed will provide you great results in maintaining consistent workouts. As you go, you will improve your flexibility in the muscles as well as the satisfaction of having successfully finished a stretching workout.

As every physical activity, the results always depend on the intensity level you are using. For this program I have listed down intensity levels, and I will explain them a bit more detailed. Intensity is controlled by the amount of pain associated with the physical activity, with a scale from 0 to 10. Light tense is scaled from 1 to 3. This means that you only stretch light enough to a point where you feel the stretch with a small light pain. Medium stretching are scaled from 4 to 6, where you should start to feel increased pain in the muscle you are stretching. Heavy stretching is scaled from 7 to 10, here you will initially experience a medium to heavy amount of pain at the start of the stretch. Do not worry, as the experienced pain will slowly evaporate as the stretching continues.

Heavy stretches provide great improvements in flexibility and strength. It is therefore important for your own success to monitor the stretch intensity and slowly move towards the fourth level. It can be very helpful to know the joint movements that each muscle can do to get the maximum stretching benefit in every muscle. With every stretch you make, try to put the joint through the full range of each motion. This will then allow for maximum stretching.

You are free to customize any given exercise in this book, which will result into more stretch combinations. Bare in mind that this book is written for beginners, and thus may seem very basic in case you are very advanced. This also means that there is only a small portion illustrated of all the available stretches out there, I want to make sure that a solid basic understanding of stretching is provided to beginners. You are encouraged to experiment with these stretches and discover more.

Try to keep making alterations in the position until you reach the desired level of the stretch by using the pain scale rating. I have tried to make the stretching program as detailed as possible, but I also tried to avoid an overload of scientific information for every stretch.

Specific instructions are giving related to time to hold the stretch and also the time to rest between each stretch you make. The number of suggested repetitions are listed to make it easier for you to understand the content of the tables. When you follow the instructions to the letter, you should notice flexibility improvements as you progress through the levels.

The program listed below are specific stretching recommendations based on my own experience as well as your individual flexibility. Should you be an absolute beginner, then I would highly recommend to stay at least four weeks on the same level before going to the next level. Try not to force it, as this will most likely end up with sports injuries which will only delay your progress more.

Level 1
Hold time: 10 to 15 seconds per stretch.
Rest time: 5 to 10 seconds between every stretch.
Repetition: 2 times.
Duration: 10 to 15 minutes per session.
Intensity scale: 1 to 3 – light pain.
Sessions: 2 to 3 times per week.

Level 2

Hold time: 15 to 20 seconds per stretch.

Rest time: 10 to 15 seconds between every stretch.

Repetition: 3 times.

Duration: 20 to 25 minutes per session.

Intensity scale: 2 to 4 – medium pain.

Sessions: 3 to 4 times per week.

Level 3

Hold time: 20 to 25 seconds per stretch.

Rest time: 15 to 20 seconds between every stretch.

Repetition: 4 times.

Duration: 30 to 35 minutes per session.

Intensity scale: 4 to 7 – medium pain.

Sessions: 4 to 5 times per week.

Level 4

Hold time: 25 to 30 seconds per stretch.

Rest time: 20 to 25 seconds between every stretch.

Repetition: 5 times.

Duration: 40 to 45 minutes per session.

Intensity scale: 8 to 10 – medium to heavy pain.

Sessions: 5 times per week.

Chapter 5: Stretching Exercises

If you are one of the many people out there who are not getting the results you want from your exercise routine, this has most likely to do that your muscle groups are too stiff. When one muscle group is stiff, it will prevent others from improving and progressing. Stated previously, doing just static stretches, where you hold your position is not necessarily the most effective approach to increase your flexibility. Another great way of stretching to create flexibility is called isolated stretching, which we have discussed in the second chapter. It involves contracting one muscle group while stretching the other. This triggers a muscular reflex that will increase your range of motion and deepen the stretch. As with all the other stretches, it does not have to take an hour per day of your time.

I have listed 6 stretches for you after your regular workout program, try to slowly progress towards doing them after every workout session. You will see improvement to your flexibility in just weeks, it will also improve both your strength and endurance in the same amount of time.

Active Pigeon Stretch
Muscles: The Piriformis

- Begin in a full push-up position, palms aligned under shoulders.
- Place left knee on the floor near shoulder with left heel by right hip.
- Lower down to forearms and bring right leg down with the top of the foot on the floor (not shown).
- Keep chest lifted to the wall in front of you, gazing down.
- If you're more flexible, bring chest down to floor and extend arms in front of you.
- Pull navel in toward spine and tighten your pelvic-floor muscles; contract right side of glutes.
- Curl right toes under while pressing ball of foot into the floor, pushing through your heel.
- Bend knee to floor and release; do 5 reps total, then switch sides and repeat.

Curve Stretch

Muscles: Lower Back

- Sit on the floor with your knees bent and place your feet about 12 inches in front of you.
- Put your interlace fingers behind both hamstrings, your elbows should be pointing out to the sides.
- Round your back, tighten the pelvic floor and pull your navel in towards your spine; focus on your belly button with the jaw pulled in. Inhale through your nose, and exhale through your mouth.
- As you exhale, draw your navel in even tighter and lift your left leg, pushing the left heel towards the wall in front of you while pulling back with your pinkie toe; at the same time, push down on your right foot.
- Return to the start position and repeat.
- Do 5 repetitions; switch sides and repeat.

Modified Cobra

Muscles: Abdominals

- Lie face down on the floor with your thumbs directly under the shoulders, legs extended with the tops of your feet on the floor.
- Tighten your pelvic floor, and tuck your hips downward as you squeeze your glutes.
- Press the shoulders down and away from your ears.
- Push through your thumbs and index your fingers as you raise your chest towards the wall in front of you.
- Relax and repeat.
- Do 5 repetitions total.

Hamstring Stretch

Muscles: Hamstrings

- Lie down faceup on the floor with your legs extended and feet flexed.
- Bend your right knee to the chest and interlace your fingers behind the hamstrings as close to your groin as possible; gaze at your chest and keep your chin down and neck long.
- Tighten the muscles of your pelvic floor and extend your leg, pushing through the heel and contracting quads.
- Return to start and repeat; do 5 repetitions.
- Repeat, turning thigh outward for 5 repetitions.
- Rest and repeat, turning thigh inward for 5 repetitions.
- Switch legs; repeat the series for a total of 15 repetitions on each leg.

Split Squat

Muscles: Quads, Calves

- Stand with your feet hip-width apart.
- Step your right foot about 12 inches in front.
- Curl the toes of your left leg; keep your weight equal between both feet. Interlace your fingers, placing your hands under the ribs; press the shoulders down away from your ears.
- Tighten the muscles of your pelvic floor; tuck your pelvis under and squeeze glutes.
- Slowly bend both knees, coming down in 3 counts; feel the stretch along the left quad.
- Press into the floor to rise back to start in 3 counts.
- Do 5 repetitions; switch legs and repeat.

Quadrupeds

Muscles: Shoulders

- Kneel on all fours with your wrists aligned under the shoulders and knees under the hips.
- Bring your forehead toward the floor and slide the pinkie edge of your left hand along the floor in front of you, keep your right palm flat on the floor.
- Press the shoulders down away from your ears and squeeze your glutes.
- Return to starting position by pushing down on your right palm and sliding your left hand back toward your shoulders.
- Do 5 repetitions; switch sides and repeat.

Chapter 6: Cooling Down

By now, you most likely know that stretching is a vital port of any workout routine. You have now learned why stretching is important and how to warm up properly to avoid injuries while stretching. Although, many people are still confused whether to stretch before or after an exercise. The short answer is: both.

Stretching before or after is not an option to choose from. I highly recommend to stretch before and after any physical activity. It is not recommended to simply stretch quickly after every exercise either, make sure to do it before and after the entire workout program.

The reason why we stretch before doing our exercises is to help prevent any possible muscle injury. This is done by lengthening our muscles and tendons by stretching them, which in turn increases your range of movement as well. Once you are done stretching your muscles, you will be able to move freely without any restriction or occurring injury. However, the reason why you should stretch after your workout program is totally different.

So why should we stretch after our workout program? After every strenuous activity, especially weightlifting, we are causing a small amount of damage to the muscles we are using and the associated soft tissues. This small amount of rips and tears in the muscles are what will force our muscles to grow when they start the process of recovery and repairing themselves. As soon as any tissue gets slightly damaged, a stronger tissue will replace it, which will often cause muscle soreness up to 2 days after your workout program. This is called Delayed Onset Muscle Soreness [DOMS]. It may happen that you do not feel the soreness immediately after your workout, however, it is a very common saying in the sports branch that you will pay for it later.

It is important to stretch after your exercises, this will help to release the tension and prevents the muscles from becoming tight. As soon as you are finished with your workout, your muscles will be warm and elastic. The post workout stretching session has given you an extra chance to loosen up your tight and perhaps even tired muscles.

However, a common mistake is to consider stretching as a cooling down. Stretching and cooling down your muscles after your workout are two very different things. Some might tell you that you should cool down first and then stretch after, while others might say that stretching can be incorporated as part of the cool down process. Make sure to understand that the whole purpose of cooling down is to help your heart rate return to normal. Your whole body, including your heart, lungs and blood flow all worked very hard to get you through your tense workout. Without a sufficient cooling down process, you will most likely feel dizzy or even slightly sick afterwards. Some people prefer to do the stretching before the cooling down, where others prefer to do it after. Should you feel urged to walk it off with a leisurely five-minute walk on the treadmill to relax your body and cool it down first, this is totally acceptable. Just make sure to not forget about the stretching part after your small walk. Because your muscles are still warm after walking you will produce the same benefits of a post-workout stretch.

Conclusion

I would like to thank you once again for downloading and reaching all the way to the end of this book about stretching exercises for beginners. Now that you have the basic knowledge of stretching exercises, I hope you have found some of the answers you were looking for about stretching, avoiding injuries, improving muscle flexibility and gaining strength.

The information I have provided to you in this book are through own experience as well as a high amount of research on the stretching topic to being able to only give you the best recommendations and suggestions out there. With this information, followed by the letter, you should be able to accomplish your maximum flexibility permitted by your body structure. Simultaneous you will also be able to develop your strength.

Finally, if you enjoyed reading this book or have any feedback suggestions, then I would kindly ask you to leave a review behind on Amazon. Should you have suggestions for a subject in the future which you want to explore further, please let me know through the review button as well. It would be greatly appreciated by the community.

Thank you very much and I wish you all the luck towards your next goal.

Dan C. Wilson

About the Author

It has been my passion and hobby to increase vitality and how to become the strongest and best version of yourself since 2009. The goals of my books are simple, it is to share powerful ideas that help us all to become stronger, healthier, more flexible in every way possible. Building strength and becoming the strongest version of yourself goes far beyond lifting heavy weights and growing muscle.

My books are all about having more vitality, flexibility, health, building better relationships, creating an attractive body, nutrition and abundance. In case you want to reach your full human potential on both mentally and physically aspect and become a strong and healthy looking person, who feels amazing every day and is respected and admired by friends, family and strangers, then you are definitely in the right place here.

It is my goal to help as many people as possible. That having said, in case I can change the life of one person and make that one person feel better and more successful in life, I have reached my goal. We are all in this together! You, me and everyone else in our community. Together we will work hard and spread the message of changing lives and make our surroundings stronger and healthier. We will create a healthier and stronger world!

Dan C. Wilson

Other Books by Dan C. Wilson

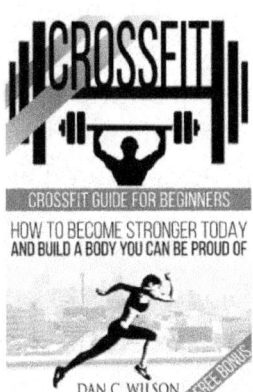

CrossFit: CrossFit Guide for Beginners – How to Become Stronger Today and Build a Body You Can Be Proud Of
by Dan C. Wilson (Author)

Find the benefits of CrossFit here! Tested and proven programs, exercises and diets to improve your flexibility, strength and conditioning.

If you would like to be fitter, stronger, more athletic, and more mobile, then CrossFit will definitely help. CrossFit is a training program that builds strength and conditioning through extremely varied and challenging workouts. Each day the workout will test a different part of your functional strength or conditioning, not specializing in one particular thing, but rather with the goal of building a body that's capable of practically anything and everything.

Much of CrossFit's growing fan base are motivated and determined with passion to continue the sport and becoming the best version of themselves, join the community and become one of the many motivated and determined people of CrossFit by starting with this   book!

This book will give you all the information you need to accomplish the maximum flexibility, strength and conditioning   permitted   by   your   body.

All the information provided to you in this book is through own experience as well as a high amount of research on the CrossFit topic for being able to only give you the best recommendations and suggestions out there. With the information of this book, you should be able to accomplish your maximum flexibility, strength and conditioning permitted by your body structure.

Take action today and make the first step towards your success by downloading this book "CrossFit: CrossFit Guide for Beginners – How to Become Stronger Today and Build a Body You Can Be Proud Of".

Preview of "CrossFit: CrossFit Guide for Beginners – How to Become Stronger Today and Build a Body You Can Be Proud Of".

Chapter 1: Explanation of CrossFit

Before we get into the more advanced part of this CrossFit book, it is important to have an idea of what CrossFit exactly is. In four words it is advertised as "the sports of fitness". It is different compared to regular fitness, as your body will be dealing with constantly varied, high-intensity functional movements. Where regular fitness is often done to gain strength and muscles, CrossFit delivers a variation of fitness which is very broad, general and inclusive. Every aspect of your body will be focused such as, stamina, strength, endurance, power, speed, agility, balance, accuracy and coordination.

The methodology and adaptations of CrossFit are individually unique. CrossFit has been aiming for years to forge a broad, general and inclusive fitness. People are prepared in the best possible way with various programs to succeed in the unknown. Through CrossFit you will build strength and conditioning through extremely, challenging and varied workouts. Your body will be tested every day during your workout with different parts of your strength and conditioning. The focus will lie on solely muscle building, instead you will build a body that is capable of practically anything. The exercises you will perform are all natural, effective and efficient to your body. Each exercise you will be performing are all equal to each other, and none of the movements are more important than the other.

A quick side note, which I would like to add is that you should try avoiding to start too quickly. It is a common problem amongst people who start a new workout program too quickly, the overly ambitious training schedule will make your body feel weak and tired. This will then result in demotivation, which often results in giving up after just a few weeks. As with everything else you start with in life, it is very important to start steady and consistent to make improvements to keep the motivation high.

Once you get a slow but steady start and you get accustomed to your new workout program, you will see improved results. It Is absolutely not necessary to start off in a very extreme way. We all know by now that the turtle can beat the rabbi, by being consistent.

Often people partner up with someone else to keep the motivation and encouragement up to workout. If you struggle with keeping the motivation high when working out on your own, then CrossFit is definitely meant for you. CrossFit is often performed in groups to keep the motivation up, and it also adds to the social aspect of going to the gym.

In case you are an absolute beginner, which is likely – as you are reading this beginners guide book, I would recommend to look for a CrossFit gym near you and try out a class for free. Do not be frightened in case you are alone or a beginner, gym classes are usually set up in different levels. Often there are introduction classes for people just like you, to get a quick overview of the basics, and getting to know each other. Once you are more experienced, you will be able to join the regular CrossFit group. No matter how experienced you are, it will be very valuable and worth your time.

The CrossFit regular classes are somewhat the same as normal fitness workout routines. A regular class will ask 45 till 60 minutes of your time, depending on the instructor. Since it is a group activity, each person will start at the same time, and the instructor will keep track and help out where needed.

The workout will always start with a dynamic warm up. This ranges from doing squats till normal stretches. The warm up routine will most likely be a bit different from what you are used to.

Once the warming up has finished, the next exercises will depend on the workout day. This is abbreviated as "WOD" in the CrossFit world, meaning "Workout Of the Day". It is here, where you will be told to do a certain amount of repetitions of a particular exercise as quickly as possible. The exercises will vary from day to day, ask your instructor about it to be more prepared for the next day!

Lastly, when the daily WOD has been finished, you will either do a cooling down as a group, or individually. This will include a certain amount of different stretches and cooling down exercises.

1.1
CrossFit Foundations

The main focus in CrossFit programs are improving your strength and conditioning. All of the CrossFit programs are designed to train your adaptational response as quickly as possible, with very broad exercises. Take in mind that CrossFit is not meant to specialize you in any way. The foundation of CrossFit started as a development to enhance an individual's competency at all physical tasks. By being part of a CrossFit community, you will be trained to perform multiple, diverse, and randomized physical challenges.

Over the years, CrossFit has proven to be effective to improve many aspects of your body. You will develop power with multiple training modalities and consistency. A common misunderstanding of CrossFit is that it is solely lifting weights while being in a group. You will be trained in gymnastics from rudimentary to advanced movements, this ranges from biking, running, swimming, rowing on short, middle, and long distances.

CrossFit is for everyone, there are no circumstances of gender, age, disability, weight or even your experience level that may reduce the safety or effectiveness of functional movement. Should you deal with any of the above mentioned circumstance, do not worry, the instructor will give you plenty of alternative exercises to get the same results. Human beings deal with body limitations, due to muscle soreness, injuries or lacking strength, it is very common for an individual to not being able to perform a particular exercise. There will always be another method to reduce the load to insignificant levels while preserving precisely the line of action of similar similar lines of actions that will prepare your body and muscles for the missing capacity.

CrossFit is meant to be safe, enjoyable and productively self-taught. Do not entirely rely on a coach or instructor, you will be stimulated to commit study and practice the basic movements to improve your experience drastically.

www.ingramcontent.com/pod-product-compliance
Lightning Source LLC
Chambersburg PA
CBHW070958180526
45168CB00003B/1201